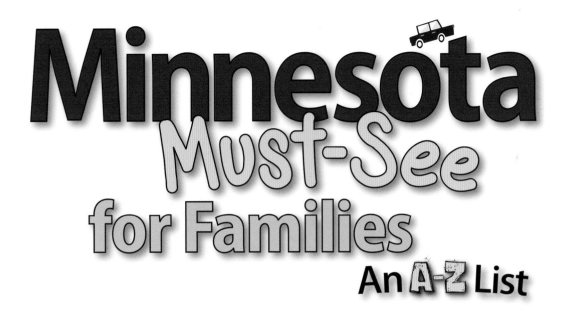

Minnesota
Must-See
for Families
An A-Z List

by Christie Gove-Berg

Adventure Publications
Cambridge, Minnesota

Dedication

For Owen, Adelyn and Annamarie, who bring me immeasurable joy.

A Note from the Author

My family is always looking for fun activities. The kids love to try new things and to visit new places. This is how we build memories and a shared history. And, yes, I am one of those Minnesotans who is always telling others why our state is the best place to live. So this book was born out of love for Minnesota and love for my family. It's a tour of the best that Minnesota has to offer, it's a scrapbook, and it's a journal of family adventures—all in one!

Edited by Ryan Jacobson
Cover and book design and illustrations by Lora Westberg

Photo credits
Peter C. Berg: 32, 48 **Yinan Chen:** front cover background **Trevor Cokley:** 46 **Peter L. Gove:** 18 main, 28 **Christie Gove-Berg:** 4, 24, 54 inset, back cover **Aaron Hautala:** front cover "C," 8 **Ryan Jacobson:** 34 **Deane Johnson:** front cover "I," 20 **Skye Marthaler:** 12 **Amy Meredith:** 36 **Minnesota Wild:** 50 **MNDNR:** 14 **National Eagle Center:** 48 main **Shutterstock:** 26 inset, 30, 40 inset **Chrissy Sorenson:** 52 **Lora Westberg:** 54 **page 44:** "Train arriving at the station," by Mac Hughes; www.flickr.com/photos/11375428@N04/14632867404/
Photo on page 42 © (2008) State of Minnesota, Department of Natural Resources, reprinted with permission

The following unaltered photos are licensed according to the Creative Commons 2.0 Attribution License, which is available here: https://creativecommons.org/licenses/by/2.0/ **page 6:** "Paul Bunyan," by Flickr User Twostoumonks; www.flickr.com/photos/twostoutmonks/635580828/ **page 10:** "Under the Lift Bridge," by Flickr User Sharon Mollerus; www.flickr.com/photos/clairity/154082270/ **page 16:** "Madhouse at Gooseberry Falls State Park," (image altered) by Flickr User m01229; www.flickr.com/photos/39908901@N06/>; www.flickr.com/photos/39908901@N06/7940528936/ **page 18 inset:** "The Minnesota History Center in St. Paul," by Flickr User Nostri-Imago, www.flickr.com/photos/nostri-imago/2873814749/ **front cover "J," page 22:** "Lichen Fear the Hand," by Flickr User bhs128; www.flickr.com/photos/bhs128/730235000/ **page 26 main:** "Common Loons," by Gary J. Wege, USFWS Midwest; www.flickr.com/photos/usfwsmidwest/4514433523/ **front cover "R," page 38:** "Old No. 1," by Flickr User Randen Pederson; www.flickr.com/photos/chefranden/4625195141/ **page 40 main:** "Split Rock Lighthouse," (image altered) by Flickr User Akshay Panday; www.flickr.com/photos/akshay012/2614232935

10 9 8 7 6 5 4 3 2

Copyright 2015 by Christie Gove-Berg
Published by Adventure Publications
820 Cleveland Street South
Cambridge, Minnesota 55008
(800) 678-7006

www.adventurepublications.net
Printed in the U.S.A.
ISBN: 978-1-59193-525-4; eISBN: 978-1-59193-518-6

Minnesota Must-See Checklist

Check off the boxes as you and your family visit each site or complete each activity.

- ☐ **A** - Agate
- ☐ **B** - Babe the Blue Ox
- ☐ **C** - Cuyuna Country
- ☐ **D** - Duluth
- ☐ **E** - Eagle Mountain (BWCAW)
- ☐ **F** - Forestville (Mystery Cave)
- ☐ **G** - Gooseberry Falls
- ☐ **H** - History Center
- ☐ **I** - Itasca State Park

- ☐ **J** - Jeffers Petroglyphs
- ☐ **K** - Kayaking
- ☐ **L** - Loons & Lady's Slippers
- ☐ **M** - Mill City Museum
- ☐ **N** - Northern Lights
- ☐ **O** - On-a-stick! (State Fair)
- ☐ **P** - Pipestone (Monument)
- ☐ **Q** - Quirky Minnesota
- ☐ **R** - Railroad

- ☐ **S** - Split Rock Lighthouse
- ☐ **T** - Tower (Soudan Mine)
- ☐ **U** - Union Depot
- ☐ **V** - Vasaloppet (Skiing)
- ☐ **W** - Wabasha (Eagle Center)
- ☐ **X** - Xcel Center (Hockey)
- ☐ **Y** - Yellow Brick Road
- ☐ **Z** - Zoo

Check out the journal pages on page 56 and the Tips for Parents on page 60.

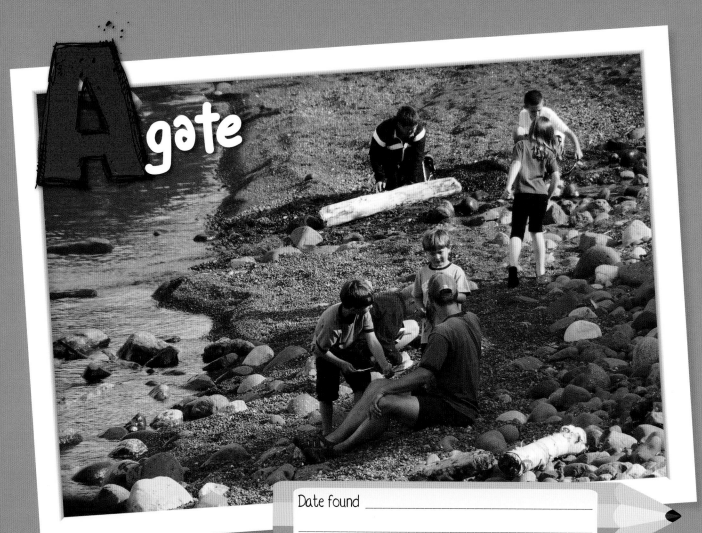

Agate

Date found _____
_____

Agate Hunting

The Lake Superior agate is the official Minnesota gemstone. Searching for these beautiful red, orange and yellow gemstones feels like a treasure hunt. Agates formed millions of years ago when minerals settled into air bubbles within recently cooled lava (liquid hot rock). The red and orange coloring in agates comes from iron, an important mineral in our state. Go with an adult and search beaches, gravel roads and even hilly fields to find an agate. Good luck hunting!

Fun Stuff:

- Go agate hunting, but be very patient. Most agates are small, like the size of a dime or a quarter.

- Start your own rock collection. Get a shoe box (or something else to keep the rocks in), and collect interesting rocks of different sizes, shapes and colors.

- Visit a rock shop. They're fun places to look at and learn about rocks and minerals.

How long did you look for agates? _____

Where did you find your favorite agate (or rock)? _____

How does it feel to find an agate? _____

_____

Babe the Blue Ox

BEMIDJI

PAUL
BUNYAN
1937

Date visited _____
_____

Paul Bunyan and Babe the Blue Ox

Legend says that Paul Bunyan was a giant lumberjack with amazing strength. He traveled throughout Minnesota many years ago with his companion: a huge blue ox named Babe. There are countless tall tales about Bunyan and Babe. For instance, it's said that they formed Minnesota's 10,000 lakes when they took a walk after a rainstorm. (The lakes are supposedly their footprints!) The state has three famous statues of Paul Bunyan: one in Brainerd, one in Bemidji and one in Akeley.

Fun Stuff:

- Ride the carnival rides at Paul Bunyan Land near Brainerd. There's also a petting zoo, a climbing wall and more. Plus, listen for Paul's statue to say your name!

- Whose shoes are bigger, yours or baby Paul Bunyan's? To discover the answer, go to the visitor center in Bemidji. You can also check out Paul's giant-sized toothbrush.

- Take a silly picture with Paul Bunyan in Akeley. You can sit in the palm of his hand.

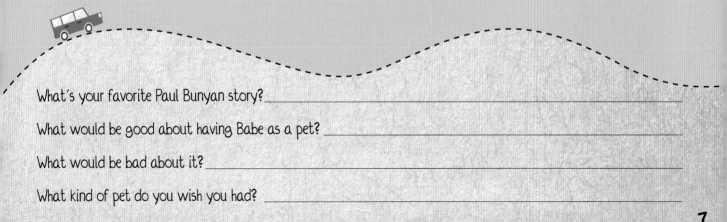

What's your favorite Paul Bunyan story?_____

What would be good about having Babe as a pet? _____

What would be bad about it? _____

What kind of pet do you wish you had? _____

Cuyuna Country

Date visited _____
_____

Cuyuna Country State Recreation Area

Located in north central Minnesota, Cuyuna Country State Recreation Area is one of Minnesota's best places for mountain biking. A few decades ago, mining companies left this area. The deep mining pits filled with water and have become large, beautiful lakes. Bike trails wind around the lakes and through the surrounding forests, making mountain biking a popular thing to do in this region. Cuyuna Country offers more than 25 miles of unpaved trails to choose from!

Fun Stuff:

- Cuyuna Country is known for its beautiful biking trails. There are different routes—from short and easy to long and challenging—for every age and skill level.

- The region's lakes are deep and clear, perfect for boating, canoeing and kayaking with parents. (But keep in mind that the lakes are very deep and very cold.)

- Bring your fishing pole and cast a line. The lakes are stocked with trout!

What trail(s) did you take?_____

How long (or how far) did you ride?_____

What did you see that was interesting? _____

What was unexpected?_____

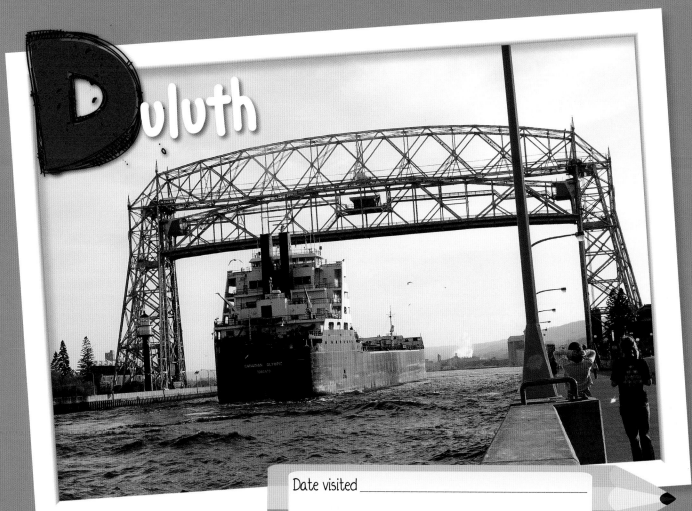

Duluth

Date visited _____

_____

Duluth, MN

Duluth sits on the western edge of Lake Superior. The city is considered the "gateway" to the North Shore—a gorgeous region of forests, trails and waterfalls. Duluth is unique because it's a seaport in the middle of the country. A ship in the Atlantic Ocean can get all the way to Duluth by traveling on special waterways. Visitors love to tour the *William A. Irvin* iron ore ship and drive over the lift bridge to Park Point Beach, a place to take a dip, climb sand dunes and hunt for rocks and driftwood.

Fun Stuff:

- Watch for big ships to come and go at Canal Park. Stroll along the shore of Lake Superior, and get your feet wet. While there, stop in at the free Maritime Museum.
- Learn about wildlife and see some huge fish at the Great Lakes Aquarium.
- At Hawk Ridge, overlooking Duluth, you can see hundreds of raptors during migration time.

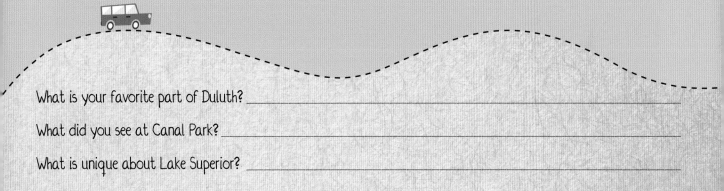

What is your favorite part of Duluth? _____

What did you see at Canal Park? _____

What is unique about Lake Superior? _____

_____

Eagle Mountain

Date visited _____
_____

Eagle Mountain of the BWCAW

Eagle Mountain is the tallest spot in Minnesota—2,301 feet above sea level. Although it's called a mountain, you don't have to climb to get to the top. Experienced hikers can follow the trails to the summit. Eagle Mountain lies within the Boundary Waters Canoe Area Wilderness (BWCAW), a protected area in northeastern Minnesota. The BWCAW is the most visited wilderness area in the United States. People go there to canoe, camp, fish, hike and swim.

Fun Stuff:

- Pitch a tent and stay a couple nights in the BWCAW. Watch for shooting stars and even the northern lights. Listen for calling loons and howling wolves.
- Look for pictographs (painted art on rock) made by American Indians who lived in this area hundreds of years ago.
- Eat a shore lunch! That means catch a fish and fry it over a campfire.

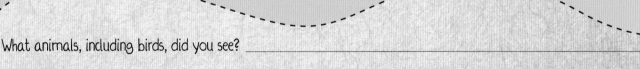

What animals, including birds, did you see? _____

Which of your five senses—hear, see, smell, taste, touch—did you use in the BWCAW and how? (For example: I SMELLED frying fish.) _____

_____

Forestville

Forestville/Mystery Cave State Park

At Forestville/Mystery Cave State Park, you can go down into the largest cave in the state! The cave's passages are 13 miles long. They were created when acidic water dissolved rock, bit by bit, over thousands of years. There is even an underground lake within the cave. The nearby town of Forestville looks like an 1800s village. You can talk with costumed actors about frontier life. The actors stay in character, so if you ask them about cars or phones, they won't know what you're talking about!

Fun Stuff:

- Go on a cave tour, and see the inside of the earth. Visitors (ages eight and up) can take a "flashlight tour" through the cave, using only a flashlight!

- Visit the historic town of Forestville. You'll live like a pioneer, feeding chickens and helping with chores. During special events, you might even get to explore the pioneer cemetery.

- Cast a fishing line into the Root River, and try to catch a big fish.

What surprised you most about the cave? _____

What surprised you most about frontier life? _____

Would you like to live in the 1800s? Why or why not? _____

_____

Gooseberry Falls

Date visited _____

_____

Gooseberry Falls State Park

A series of waterfalls that flow toward Lake Superior, Gooseberry Falls is located in the popular Gooseberry Falls State Park, the waterfalls are arguably the most beautiful in the state. They are easy to get to and fun to play around—with rocks, hiking trails and pools of water. On the shore of Lake Superior, a short hike away, there's an area of ancient lava rock called "Picnic Flow" because it's a perfect place for a picnic. This is a great example of what happens when lava hardens.

Fun Stuff:

- Explore the pools between the waterfalls. Although the rocks are slippery, some people like to get in the water.

- Hike to Agate Beach. Have a picnic and wade in the river. Chances are good that you'll find some nice agates to look at, too. (But don't keep them. At state parks, collecting is illegal.)

- Bike the Gitchi-Gami paved trail. You're only eight miles from Split Rock Lighthouse.

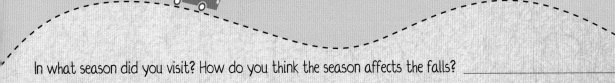

In what season did you visit? How do you think the season affects the falls? _____

_____

What did you see and hear? _____

How wet did you get?_____

17

History Center

Planting season is short. Let's get plowing!

You need a friend to plow.

Date visited _____
_____

Minnesota History Center

The Minnesota History Center in Saint Paul is packed full of fun exhibits about the culture, weather and history of our great state. If you love Minnesota, this is the place for you! There are many hands-on activities where visitors can play and learn. You'll find something new every time you visit. Be an ox, or a pioneer farmer, and plow your field. Enjoy the steps, slides and tunnels of the grain elevator play area. It's a perfect place to let out some energy!

Fun Stuff:

- Here comes a tornado! Quick, get into the cellar of a 1960s home. The wind screams around you, and a tree falls near the cellar, shattering a window.
- Take a ride in a World War II plane. It bounces, bumps and finally crashes behind enemy lines. During the ride, you'll also hear the stories of the survivors.
- Pretend you're an iron ore miner. Put down some dynamite and blow up the stone walls.

What was your favorite part of the museum? _____

What was the most interesting thing you learned? _____

What do you like best about Minnesota? Would it make a good museum exhibit? _____

_____

Itasca State Park

HERE 1475 FT
ABOVE
THE OCEAN
THE MIGHTY
MISSISSIPPI
BEGINS
TO FLOW
ON ITS
WINDING WAY
2552 MILES
TO THE
GULF OF
MEXICO

Date visited _____
_____

Itasca State Park

Itasca State Park is Minnesota's oldest state park and is a fun place for families to visit. The mighty Mississippi River starts as a small stream there, and the water from this stream ultimately travels more than 2,000 miles, all the way to the Gulf of Mexico! The park has even more to offer. Rent a boat and get out on Lake Itasca. Bring a bike and hit the park's paved trails. Pile into the car and take Wilderness Drive, a 10-mile trip through the park's most scenic areas.

Fun Stuff:

- Wade across the Mississippi River, and play in water that will travel to the ocean! (You can also cross on a log bridge if you want to keep your feet dry.)
- Visit the Indian burial mounds and the pioneer cemetery. They're interesting and historical!
- To get a good view of the park, you can climb the Aiton Heights Lookout Tower. It's a tower that was used to watch for forest fires, and it's 100 feet tall!

What words would you use to describe the Headwaters of the Mississippi River?_____

_____

What did you discover about Itasca State Park? _____

What wildlife did you see? _____

Jeffers Petroglyphs

Date visited _____
_____

Jeffers Petroglyphs

Imagine a time, thousands of years ago, when buffalo roamed the land and the sun set over waving hills of prairie grasses. Long ago, American Indians created pictures by carving them into stone. At the Jeffers Petroglyphs in southwest Minnesota, you can see some of those ancient pictures (called petroglyphs). Surprisingly, the best time to see them is just after sunrise or just before sunset. The angle of the soft light makes the pictures in the rock easier to recognize.

Fun Stuff:

- Find the petroglyphs. You can hike alone with your family, or a guide will show you exactly where the petroglyphs are located.
- Learn about American Indians by exploring the visitor center and taking part in fun programs.
- Special programs are occasionally available. You can learn to throw a spear at a buffalo target, start a fire without matches or make an arrowhead.

What petroglyphs did you see (buffalo, arrows, turtles, etc.)? _____

How did the American Indians carve the petroglyphs? _____

Why do you think they made these pictures?_____

What's your favorite way to make art (drawing, painting, coloring, etc.)?_____

Kayaking

Date experienced _____
_____

Kayaking or Canoeing

Kayaking or canoeing is a great way to experience a lake or river. Kayaks are easy to paddle alone; canoes are good options for two or three people. Either way, you can explore the shallow parts of lakes and rivers that bigger boats cannot reach. (Wear a life jacket, and go with an adult.) Paddling is just one way to enjoy our Minnesota lakes and rivers. Your family might also swim, fish, float, water ski and more! Listen for nature sounds: birds singing, loons calling and trees blowing in the wind.

Fun Stuff:

- What's more fun than kayaking or canoeing? Do it on a camping trip!
- Have you ever been fishing? There's nothing quite like pulling a fish out of the water! Experienced paddlers sometimes fish right from their kayak or canoe.
- Try paddleboarding. Stand on a special board, similar to a surf board, and dip a long paddle into the water to move.

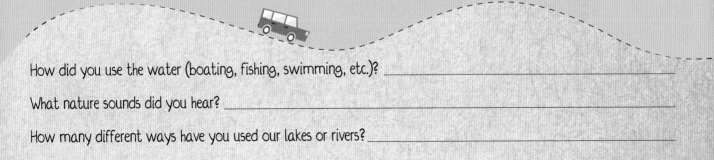

How did you use the water (boating, fishing, swimming, etc.)? _____

What nature sounds did you hear? _____

How many different ways have you used our lakes or rivers? _____

_____

25

Loons & Lady's Slippers

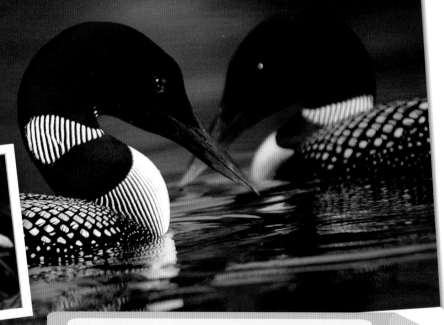

Date seen _____
_____

Common Loons and Showy Lady's Slippers

Have you ever heard a loon's call at night? It's a wild, wonderful—and slightly spooky—sound! The Common Loon is the Minnesota state bird and a symbol of the Minnesota wilderness. Loons are large birds that swim fast and dive deep. Our state flower is the Showy Lady's Slipper. It's a beautiful pink and white type of orchid that grows one to two feet tall. Lady's slippers are protected in Minnesota, so when you find one, take a picture. It's illegal to pick them.

Fun Stuff:

- Take pictures! Practice photographing the loons and lady's slippers that you see. (Maybe you can enter your pictures in a local contest, such as at a county fair.)
- Listen for the loon call. Loons have four different cries, but the tremolo or "crazy laugh" is best known. During summer, you can hear it at night on many Minnesota lakes.
- Look for lady's slippers near bogs and swamps. They bloom in late June and early July.

What did you see (color, size, etc.)? _____

_____

How did you find it? _____

Where did you see it? _____

Mill City Museum

Date visited _____
_____

Mill City Museum

The Mill City Museum in downtown Minneapolis makes flour fun! The museum focuses on the role of flour milling in the history of Minneapolis, but that's not all. Learn about flour dust and its potential to catch fire. Find out how the river helped power the mill. Discover why Minneapolis was nicknamed "Mill City" when people came here to be near the flour mill. Check out the original exploded mill ruins, the train shed and original railroad tracks from the 1800s.

Fun Stuff:

- Ride up the "flour tower" freight elevator, and check out the amazing views of Saint Anthony Falls and the Stone Arch Bridge.

- Watch an example of a mill explosion in the exhibit hall. You might want to cover your ears!

- Sample a tasty baked treat in the baking lab.

What did you learn about flour mills?_____

_____

What was your favorite part of the museum? _____

What is your favorite food that has flour in it? _____

Northern Lights

Date seen _____
_____

Northern Lights

If you should ever look into the night sky and see colorful moving lights, you're not dreaming. It's probably the northern lights! These beautiful colors in the sky happen when energized particles from the sun crash into atoms of nitrogen and oxygen in the earth's atmosphere. The northern lights are also called the aurora borealis. If all nights were clear and cloudless, the aurora could be seen in Minnesota about 100 nights per year. The aurora is usually green, but sometimes it's red or purple.

Fun Stuff:

- Go camping in a rural area. Without city lights, it's much easier to see the aurora and other stuff in the sky.
- Bring a telescope, and look at the stars. Find the North Star. (It's on the Little Dipper, at the end of the handle.) Can you find the Big Dipper, too?
- Visit a planetarium to see all sorts of amazing things in the night sky.

Where were you when you saw the aurora? _____

What color was it? _____

Did you stay up late or get up in the middle of the night? _____

What constellations did you see? _____

31

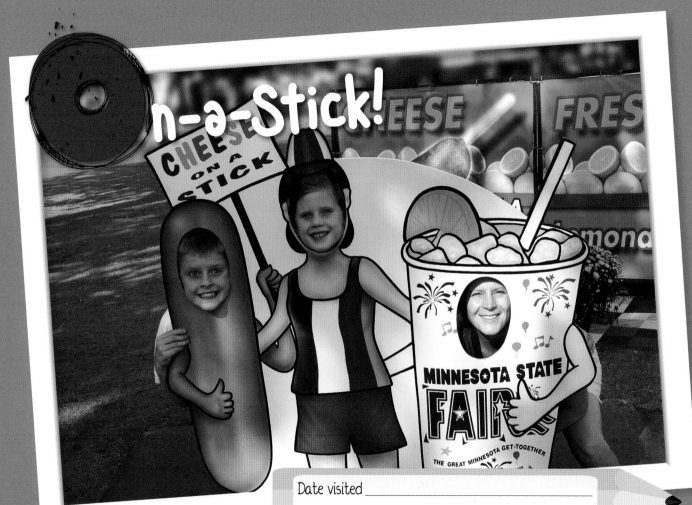

On-a-Stick!

Date visited _____
_____

Minnesota State Fair

"On-a-stick" is the way much of the food is offered at the Great Minnesota Get-together, our state fair. The Minnesota State Fair is the second largest in the country. The first food on a stick was the Pronto Pup (like a corn dog). There's so much to see and do at the fair: food, art, rides, music, animals and more! Make sure to check out the Princess Kay of the Milky Way butter sculptures. Each official state fair princess gets her likeness carved into a giant hunk of butter, and you can watch it happen!

Fun Stuff:

- Eat! From cheese curds and mini-donuts to alligator-on-a-stick and bacon dipped in chocolate, there's something for everyone.
- Grab a burlap sack, and ride the waves of the Giant Slide—a popular attraction at the fair.
- Go to the "Miracle of Birth" barn, where a baby animal might be born right in front of you!

What's your favorite thing about the fair?_____

Which fair foods do you like the most? _____

What's the weirdest thing you tasted at the fair? _____

If you had a giant hunk of butter, what would you carve into it? _____

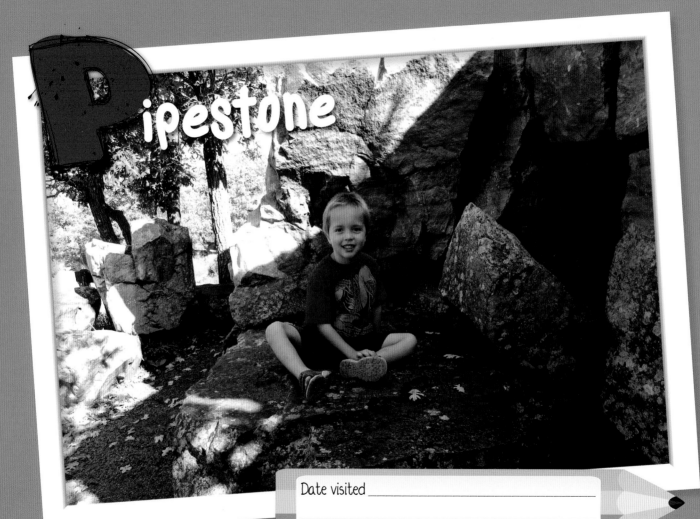

Pipestone

Date visited _____
_____

Pipestone National Monument

For thousands of years, American Indians met at the area we now call Pipestone National Monument to declare war, make peace and trade. This site in southwest Minnesota is still sacred to Native Americans who quarry (remove from the ground) the Catlinite stone, or Pipestone, a reddish rock used to make peace pipes. The American Indians smoked from the pipes as a way to seal their agreements, believing that the smoke would carry prayers to their god, the Great Spirit.

Fun Stuff:

- Explore the hiking trail. It's less than a mile long, but you'll get to walk over huge rock formations and beside a beautiful waterfall.
- At the gift shop, you'll see many amazing carvings made from Pipestone. Chances are good that an American Indian will be there, carving something new and answering your questions.
- Learn more about American Indians by viewing the visitor center's exhibits—and a movie.

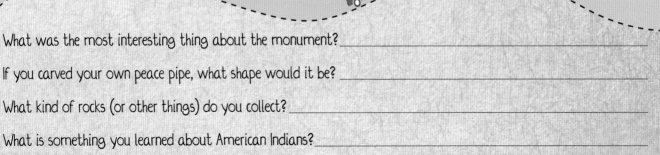

What was the most interesting thing about the monument?_____

If you carved your own peace pipe, what shape would it be? _____

What kind of rocks (or other things) do you collect?_____

What is something you learned about American Indians?_____

35

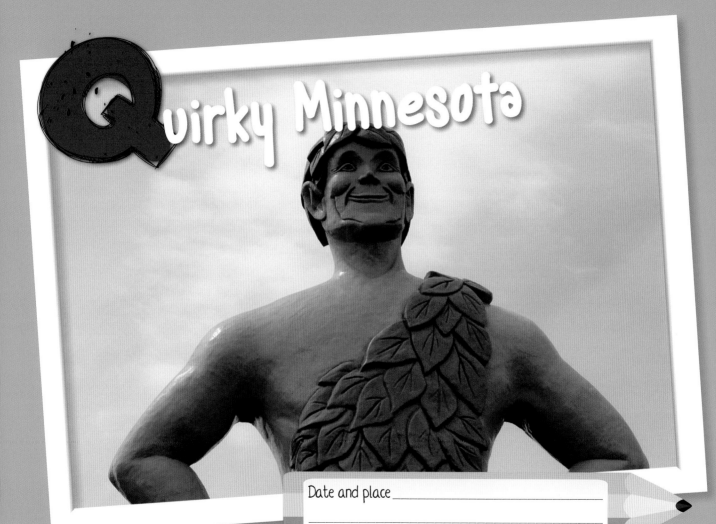

Quirky Minnesota

Date and place _____
_____

Quirky Minnesota

Minnesotans are adventurous nature-lovers, but we're also quirky—silly, funny and a little odd. There are many quirky things to see across our state, places that will make you say "What?" and "Why?" You could visit the Jolly Green Giant in Blue Earth. Or you could tour the museum in Austin entirely devoted to SPAM, meat that's sold in a can. If you see a silly, funny or odd attraction, then you'll know that you've experienced Quirky Minnesota!

Fun Stuff:

- Eat some "Spamples" in the gift store of the SPAM museum in Austin. You can taste SPAM with bacon, SPAM with cheese, SPAM with jalapeno and more!

- Visit the Big Ole statue in Alexandria. Big Ole is a huge Viking.

- Why would someone make a ball of twine the size of a car? Who knows, but you can see it in the town of Darwin.

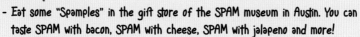

What was the quirkiest thing about the place you visited? _____

_____

Have you tried SPAM? If so, write three words to describe it. _____

What's a funny, weird or quirky thing about your family? _____

Railroad

Date visited _____
_____

The Duluth Depot

Some of the country's early railroad tracks were built in Minnesota as a way to move grains, potatoes, iron ore and wood to other parts of the US. Today, Minnesota is crisscrossed with railroad tracks. At the Lake Superior Railroad Museum, part of the Duluth Depot, you can see huge trains and learn how the railroad industry helped to shape northern Minnesota. Explore the Mallet Steam Locomotive, sit in the engineer's seat, and imagine driving this big train.

Fun Stuff:

- Take a train ride along the shore of Lake Superior on the North Shore Scenic Railroad. There are also special rides for every season.
- Check out the Lake Superior Railroad Museum's model railroad displays and working trains.
- At the Jackson Street Roundhouse in Saint Paul, you can see a genuine operating roundhouse turntable, one of the last of its kind in the whole country.

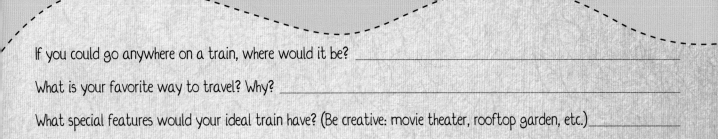

If you could go anywhere on a train, where would it be? _____

What is your favorite way to travel? Why? _____

What special features would your ideal train have? (Be creative: movie theater, rooftop garden, etc.) _____

_____

Split Rock Lighthouse

Date visited _____

_____

Split Rock Lighthouse

In 1905, a huge storm wrecked many ships along the rocky shores of Lake Superior. During that storm, some ship captains couldn't see the cliffs, which caused them to crash. Split Rock Lighthouse was built at Stony Point to help ships navigate more safely. It was used until 1969, when most ships began using radar for navigation. Split Rock Lighthouse has since become one of the most famous historic landmarks in Minnesota and a popular site on the North Shore of Lake Superior.

Fun Stuff:

- When you visit, climb the stairs all the way to the top of the lighthouse, and see the original light that shone out over the dark waters of Lake Superior.

- Walk through the original lighthouse keeper's home, and see how he lived.

- If you want to see the beacon lit, visit on November 10. The lighthouse shines in memory of all the shipwrecks of the Great Lakes, most notably the *Edmund Fitzgerald*.

Would you like to be a lighthouse keeper? Why or why not? _____

_____

If you were a captain, what would you name your ship? _____

Do you think shipwrecks are creepy or cool? Why? _____

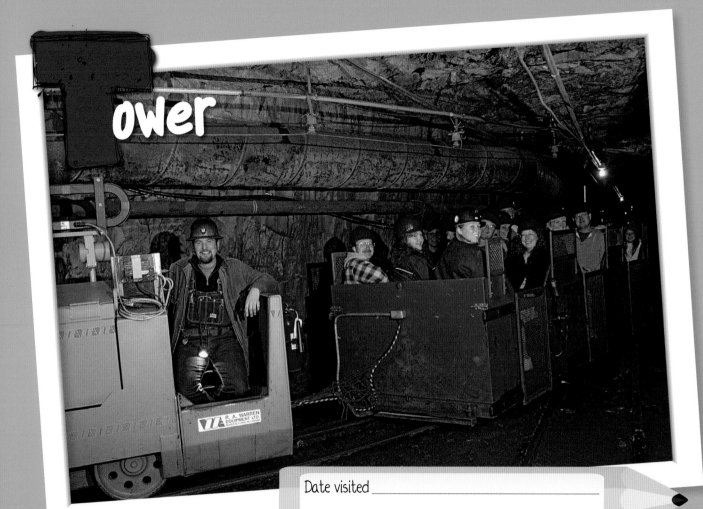

ower

Date visited_____
_____

Lake Vermillion-Soudan Underground Mine State Park near Tower, MN

Do you want to go underground and see a real iron ore mine? If so, then Lake Vermillion-Soudan Underground Mine State Park, near Tower, is the place for you! Put on a hard hat and learn about the importance of mining to Minnesota. Original miners worked in semi-darkness, using steam drills to extract the hard iron ore. Then mules that lived in the mine pulled the ore carts out. Iron ore was made into steel and was used to make cars and buildings, as well as planes and ships for World War II.

Fun Stuff:

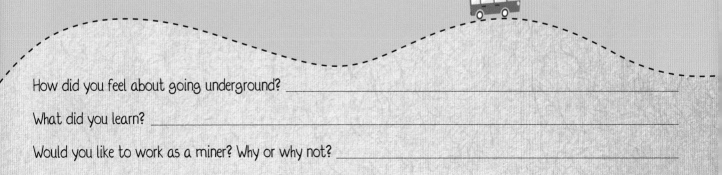

- Ride an elevator down a half mile underground, then travel in a mine car to see how iron ore miners worked. If you ask, they might turn off the lights!

- Explore above ground. Learn all about what miners did at the drill shop, crusher house and engine house.

- Take a hike outside, peer into abandoned mine pits, and check out the Soudan iron formation.

How did you feel about going underground? _____

What did you learn? _____

Would you like to work as a miner? Why or why not? _____

_____

Union Depot

Date visited _____
_____

Union Depot

In the early 1900s, the Union Depot in Saint Paul was one of the nation's great train stations. It has been restored to its original beauty with tall ceilings, wall carvings and natural skylights. Take a walk through this busy transportation hub, where you can ride the light rail, take a city bus, catch a train to Chicago or rent a bike to explore along the river. Make sure to visit the waiting area at the back of the building to watch trains pass by.

Fun Stuff:

- Ride the light rail to Minneapolis. The "Green Line" starts at the Union Depot and goes all the way to Target Field.
- Have a picnic at the Railview Picnic Area, where you can see trains roll by!
- Visit the Twin City Model Railroad Museum at 652 Transfer Road in Saint Paul to see railroad models of Minneapolis and Saint Paul.

What did you enjoy most about the Union Depot? _____

Do you prefer busy places with lots of people or quiet places without many people? Why? _____

_____

What do you like most about visiting new places? _____

Vasaloppet

Date experienced _____

_____

Vasaloppet

Cross country skiing is one of Minnesota's most popular winter sports. Each year, the east-central town of Mora hosts the Vasaloppet ski race. The Mora Vasaloppet is a sister race to a 90-kilometer (56-mile) race that takes place in Sweden. In fact, the prize for winning the Mora Vasaloppet is a trip to ski in the Swedish Vasaloppet! Skiing is a great way to enjoy the cold, snowy winter. Other fun winter activities include broomball, ice fishing, ice skating, sledding, snowboarding and snowshoeing.

Fun Stuff:

- Ski the Mora Miniloppet for kids. Or sign your parents up for the big race!

- Go on a dog sledding adventure. In northern Minnesota, there are places that offer this winter experience of a lifetime. Fair warning: it's pretty expensive.

- Try a new winter sport this year—maybe ice skating, broomball or downhill skiing? Get out there and enjoy winter!

What winter activities have you tried? _____

Which is your favorite? _____

What winter activities would you still like to try? _____

Which Minnesota season is your favorite? _____

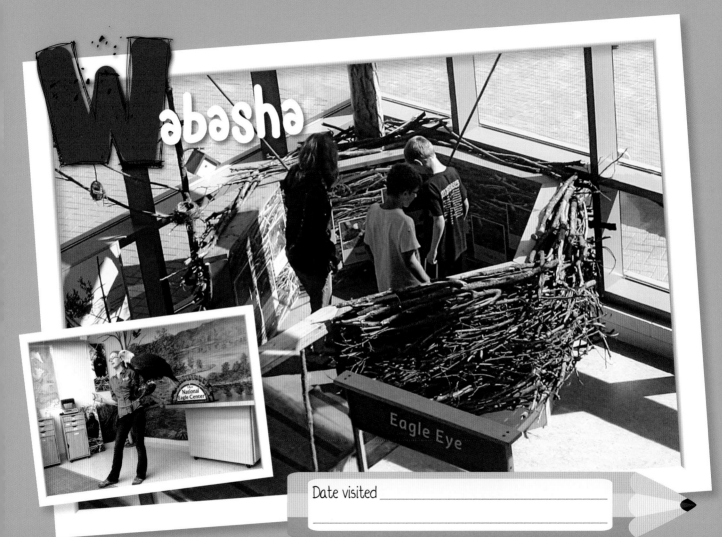

Wabasha

Eagle Eye

National Eagle Center

Date visited _____
_____

The National Eagle Center

The Bald Eagle is our national emblem (or symbol), but did you know the National Eagle Center is located right here in Minnesota? If you want to see eagles, come to Wabasha in the southeastern part of the state. The National Eagle Center is on the Mississippi River, and during summer and winter migrations, Bald and Golden Eagles gather along this stretch of water. The fast current keeps the river from freezing, so eagles are able to catch fish in the open water.

Fun Stuff:

- Attend the eagle program at the National Eagle Center. You'll get to see one of the resident eagles up close. You might even get to watch as it's fed!

- Bring your binoculars and count how many eagles you can see along the river.

- Check out the big eagle nest on the center's main floor, and test your grip strength compared to an eagle's. Can you hold onto prey as tightly as a Bald Eagle does?

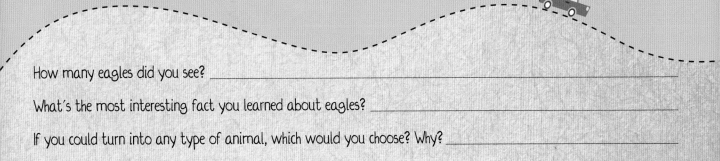

How many eagles did you see? _____

What's the most interesting fact you learned about eagles? _____

If you could turn into any type of animal, which would you choose? Why? _____

_____

Xcel Energy Center

Date visited _____

_____

Xcel Energy Center

The Xcel Energy Center in Saint Paul is the home of Minnesota's professional hockey team, the Minnesota Wild. The Xcel is also where the state high school hockey tournament is played each year. The tournament often draws more than 100,000 fans in total attendance! Minnesota is known as "the State of Hockey" because the sport is so popular. It isn't just played in arenas, though. People across the state like to play pond hockey and friendly neighborhood games, just for the fun of it.

Fun Stuff:

- Go to a local hockey game and cheer for your team, or attend a game at the Xcel and root for the Minnesota Wild.

- Visit the US Hockey Hall of Fame in Eveleth. Learn about this popular sport, and see the giant hockey stick on-site, along with a 700-pound hockey puck!

- The Xcel is also a great place to see a concert, show or special performance.

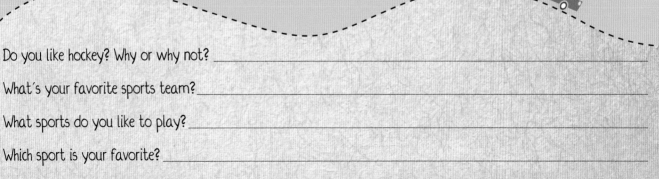

Do you like hockey? Why or why not? _____

What's your favorite sports team? _____

What sports do you like to play? _____

Which sport is your favorite? _____

Yellow Brick Road

Date visited _____
_____

Judy Garland Museum

"Follow the Yellow Brick Road" was a popular song in the 1939 movie, *The Wizard of Oz*. Judy Garland, who was born in Grand Rapids, Minnesota, played Dorothy, the girl who traveled to Oz and faced off against the Wicked Witch of the West. Now, Grand Rapids is home to the Judy Garland Museum. See memorabilia from Garland's life and from the movie. But you won't find Dorothy's ruby slippers there. They were stolen in 2005 and haven't yet been found!

Fun Stuff:

- Take a walk through Judy Garland's childhood home. Then find the "horse of a different color" carriage. It is an actual carriage that appeared in the movie.
- In the attached children's museum, be a paleontologist and dig for dinosaur bones!
- Dress up and become a townsperson in the pretend town. There's a fire station, a medical clinic, a grocery store and more.

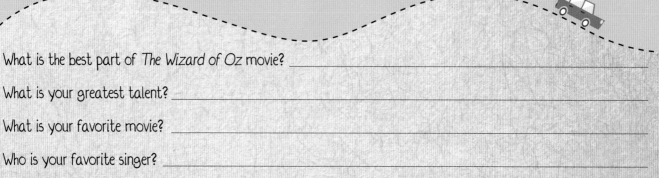

What is the best part of *The Wizard of Oz* movie? _____

What is your greatest talent? _____

What is your favorite movie? _____

Who is your favorite singer? _____

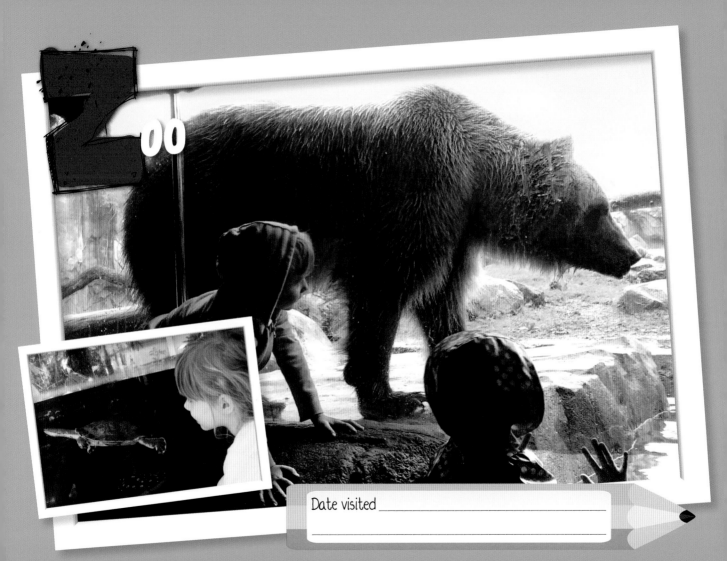

Zoo

Date visited _____
_____

Zoo

Como Park Zoo and Conservatory in Saint Paul and the Minnesota Zoo in Apple Valley offer great wildlife viewing opportunities! At Como, visit "Gorilla Forest," the largest all-mesh gorilla enclosure in North America. At the Minnesota Zoo, you can watch everything from bears to leopards to wild boars at Russia's Grizzly Coast. Zoos are great places to see exotic animals that you might never have seen before and to learn the value of wildlife and our natural world.

Fun Stuff:

- At Como, check out the "Polar Bear Odyssey" to see these animals up close.
- The Marjorie McNeely Conservatory is filled with pretty flowers and plants.
- Touch a shark and see large fish and stingrays at the Minnesota Zoo's "Discovery Bay."
- Test your knowledge of frog sounds at the start of the Minnesota Zoo's "Minnesota Trail."

What was your favorite animal at the zoo? Why? _____

What was the best part of your trip to the zoo? _____

Why do you think zoos are important? _____
_____

all about us

Write the names and ages of all your family members: _____
_____

What are your favorite things to do in Minnesota? _____
_____

What are your favorite Minnesota places to visit? _____
_____

What is the best trip you have taken? _____
_____

What's the funniest thing that ever happened on a trip? _____
_____

If you could travel anywhere in the world together, where would you go? Why? _____
_____

Create your own Minnesota must-see entry

Our family's must-see place is _____

Why is this place special or important to you and your family? _____

_____

What's your favorite thing about this place? _____

_____

Would other families like this place? Why or why not? _____

_____

Write a poem or draw a picture that reminds you of this must-see place:

journal

Tips for Parents

Agates: Cardboard egg cartons are great for storing and keeping special rocks. With a strip of construction paper glued onto the lid, kids can decorate the carton and/or label the rocks below.

Babe the Blue Ox (and Paul Bunyan): Paul Bunyan Land east of Brainerd feels like an old-fashioned county fair with a petting zoo, climbing wall, rides and an old town. It's great fun based on Minnesota history and folklore, and it's probably best for kids under the age of 12.

The 120-mile Paul Bunyan Bike Trail stretches from Brainerd to Bemidji. There are campsites and hotels along the way. You can bike from one Paul to another on the longest paved trail in Minnesota.

Cuyuna Country State Recreation Area: Some of the trails are more challenging, but you can find kid-friendly routes by using the state park's bike trail map, found at the visitor center. Remember to wear helmets!

Note: Minnesota is one of the most bike-friendly states in the country. Search online for a trail near you, and bike with the whole family.

Duluth: The Lakewalk, a widely paved sidewalk along Lake Superior, starts at Canal Park and is a fun way to burn some energy. It is a one-mile walk to the Fitger's Brewery Complex, where you can do a little shopping, grab a bite to eat and then walk back.

The Maritime Museum is free and will have free copies of *The Duluth Shipping News*, a daily list of which ships are coming through the canal. Of course, it's also a neat museum filled with shipwreck info and a movie with a focus on the *Edmund Fitzgerald*.

Take a drive up Seven Bridges Road, through the woods and along a stretch of beautiful Skyline Parkway. Stop at Enger Tower Park and climb the stone tower for an amazing view of Duluth.

Eagle Mountain (and the Boundary Waters Canoe Area Wilderness): Camping inside the BWCAW can be daunting for families with small children. For a great introduction, stay at a campsite at the edge of the Boundary Waters, and take day trips in with a canoe. Your family will experience the beauty of the BWCAW without needing to haul too much gear or portaging. Bring your binoculars; eagles and other wildlife are plentiful.

Forestville/Mystery Cave State Park: There are many different cave tours available, so check the website (www.dnr.state.mn.us/mysterycave/index.html) for tour descriptions and times. Older kids and cave lovers may prefer to take a more rugged or challenging tour. Bring warm clothes and sturdy shoes because the cave is always 50 degrees—in summer and winter. Flash photography is allowed in the cave.

Check the Historic Forestville town schedule before you go. It's worth a trip to see how Minnesota used to be in the late 1800s.

Tips for Parents (continued)

Gooseberry Falls State Park: You can bike the Gitchi-Gami State Trail from Gooseberry Falls State Park to Split Rock Lighthouse. It is a paved but hilly eight-mile ride each way, with some of the trail right alongside the lake.

History Center: There is a café on-site if you need to feed your crew. The Minnesota Historical Society is housed here, as well, and their files and information are available for the public to explore. Try looking up your ancestors!

Itasca State Park: This state park has tons of different ways to stay overnight. You can camp or stay in an RV. There is a youth hostel. There are individual cabins for rent, and there is a lodge with heating and air conditioning. The park also rents motorized boats, paddleboats, paddleboards, kayaks, canoes, bikes and snowshoes.

Jeffers Petroglyphs: Check the Minnesota Historical Society's website (http://sites.mnhs.org/historic-sites/jeffers-petroglyphs) to learn about the many unique programs related to American Indian traditions and cultures. Programs include playing traditional American Indian games, learning to throw a spear, making an arrowhead, finding constellations while lying on a buffalo pelt in the prairie, tasting American Indian foods and more.

Go with a guide to see the petroglyphs because they carry a special contraption that allows for easier viewing.

Kayaking: It's easy to learn how to kayak, and it's a pollution-free way to explore our amazing Land of 10,000 Lakes. The Minnesota DNR has a series of free programs, called "I Can Paddle," that helps people learn how to kayak. Check it out online at www.dnr.state.mn.us/state_parks/can_paddle.html. The parks also have "I Can!" programs for fishing, camping, climbing and mountain biking.

Loons & Lady's Slippers: Loons prefer clear, cool water, generally on lakes in the upper half of the state. Loons are at risk for lead poisoning because they eat fish whole. Switching to non-lead fishing tackle is a good way to help keep loons (and other animals) safe.

Mill City Museum: This museum was built within the walls of the ruined flour mill, so walk through the courtyard at the back of the building to see the original brickwork and limestone walls. In the summer, there's a great farmers' market next door. Plus, Gold Medal Park has a lot of green space for kids to run. You can also walk over the Stone Arch Bridge to see Saint Anthony Falls up close.

Northern Lights: Aurora activity peaks in April/May and October/November. Check online; there are many websites that try to predict high aurora activity due to sunspots and solar energy flares.

On-a-stick (Minnesota State Fair): Younger kids will love "Little Farm Hands" on Machinery Hill. They get to dress like a farmer, feed the animals, harvest crops and then sell their goods at a farmers' market in exchange for a free snack!

Tips for Parents (continued)

Pipestone: Only people of American Indian heritage have the right to quarry the Pipestone. Interesting fact: For American Indians, the color of the stone is thought to represent the blood of their ancestors.

Quirky Minnesota: Many cities have their own quirky statues: large loons, big fish, pelicans, etc. Go ahead and find your own quirky place and note that in the book.

Railroad (Duluth Depot): In December, consider a ride on the "Christmas City Express" to get in the holiday spirit. You can also attend "Night Trains" at the Twin City Model Railroad Museum. All the model trains are decked out in Christmas lights!

Split Rock Lighthouse: At the visitor center, check out the shipping and shipwreck displays. Plus, a movie details the story of building Split Rock Lighthouse and focuses on how families survived while living there.

Tower (Lake Vermillion-Soudan Underground Mine State Park): There is a large underground physics lab in the mine where "dark matter" is being studied. Older kids might enjoy learning about what they are studying deep under the ground.

The mine tour is 90 minutes and is ADA accessible. People with claustrophobia may have trouble with the ride down the mine elevator, but once you get to the bottom, it opens into a huge cavern.

Union Depot: The Amtrak "Empire Builder" train departs from the Depot. You can ride a train from Minneapolis to Chicago, or go all the way to Seattle, Washington.

Union Depot is a block from the Saint Paul Farmer's Market. Visit on a weekend morning to pick up some locally grown fruits, veggies, flowers and more.

Vasaloppet: There are many different races at the Mora Vasaloppet. Check out all the different options online (www.vasaloppet.us). Minnesota has more than 1,490 miles (2,400 kilometers) of groomed trails, so look online and find a trail near you!

Wabasha (National Eagle Center): March is a great month to visit the eagle center because hundreds of migrating eagles gather along the river. Regardless of when you visit, there are always daily eagle shows and three or four live Bald Eagles to see up close.

Xcel Energy Center: Make your kids laugh: The first hockey puck, used during outdoor pickup games in the 1800s, was reportedly made of frozen cow dung.

Tips for Parents (continued)

Yellow Brick Road (Judy Garland Museum): The Judy Garland Museum isn't the only landmark dedicated to a famous Minnesotan. Other places worth visiting include the following:

- Laura Ingalls Wilder Museum in Walnut Grove, MN. Visit the location of Laura's dugout home. On select summer weekends, see one of the "Wilder Pageants," an outdoor play based on Laura's life.

- Charles Lindbergh Historic Site in Little Falls, MN. Ride in a flight simulator and pretend you're the first to cross the ocean in a plane.

- F. Scott Fitzgerald was born in Saint Paul, MN. The Minnesota Historical Society hosts walking tours of his childhood neighborhood.

- Bob Dylan was born in Duluth, MN, and lived in Hibbing, MN, while growing up.

Como Park Zoo and Conservatory: The Como Park Zoo is located in Saint Paul and has plenty of neat animals, plus an indoor conservatory full of tropical plants—a good place to visit on a cold winter day! The conservatory will sometimes have a Showy Lady's Slipper in bloom during the early summer months. Go and see our state flower and check off the letter "L" for Ladyslipper. Como Town is a family-friendly amusement park next to Como Park Zoo. With 18 rides and attractions, it's a fun place to play after touring the zoo.

Minnesota Zoo: Get a daily schedule when you arrive. You can watch penguin feedings, the tropical reef dive show, the "world of birds" show and other special presentations throughout the day. There are a lot of food choices in a variety of locations at the zoo, so it's easy to grab a quick bite to eat. During the summer, stay for a Music in the Zoo concert—some are geared towards families/kids.

Other information: Consider buying a membership to the Minnesota Historical Society. A one-year family membership is very affordable and will get you into 26 historic sites, including Split Rock Lighthouse, Mill City Museum, Historic Forestville, the Minnesota History Center and Jeffers Petroglyphs (all in this book).

Also consider buying a Minnesota state park vehicle sticker. This permit allows for unlimited visits to all 75 Minnesota state parks and recreation areas for a full year from the month of purchase—and it costs less than taking the family out to dinner! Sites in this book include Cuyuna Country State Recreation Area, Forestville/Mystery Cave State Park, Gooseberry Falls State Park, Itasca State Park, Lake Vermillion-Soudan Underground Mine State Park and Split Rock Lighthouse State Park.

About the Author

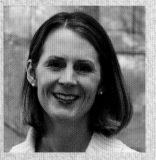

Christie Gove-Berg was born and raised in Minnesota and is bringing up her three children here, as well. With the belief that family adventures enhance family connectedness, she wrote *Minnesota Must-See for Families* to encourage kids and their parents to go exploring. Minnesota is full of amazing parks, cultural destinations and fun activities for all seasons. This book encourages kids to document their experiences in writing, so families can reflect on them for years to come.

Christie has two other published books. Her first book, *Esther the Eaglet: A True Story of Rescue and Rehabilitation*, is a children's picture book that was written in collaboration with the Raptor Center at the University of Minnesota. Her second raptor book, *Maggie the One-Eyed Peregrine Falcon: A True Story of Rescue and Rehabilitation*, was written in collaboration with the Wildlife Center of Virginia.

Christie has been a member of the Forest Lake Writers' Workshop for nine years. Her perfect day includes her family, a picnic lunch and kayaking on the Saint Croix River.

Acknowledgments

To my loving grandparents: Willard & Denise Gove and Vernon & Nona Nash.

To the hard-working people at Adventure Publications for their dedication to the art of publishing and for believing in me.

To the members of the Forest Lake Writers' Workshop for being a source of inspiration and support. I am lucky to call you my friends.

To those who work to preserve green spaces, clean waters, American Indian traditions, immigrant stories, and the culture and history of Minnesota. Thank you.